Juicing for Beginners

Learn How to Juice for Weight Loss & Health Benefits If You Have Never Juiced Before!

by Olivia Rogers

Copyright © 2017 By Olivia Rogers
All rights reserved. No part of this book may be reproduced in any form without permission in writing from the author. No part of this publication may be reproduced or transmitted in any form or by any means, mechanic, electronic, photocopying, recording, by any storage or retrieval system, or transmitted by email without the permission in writing from the author and publisher.
For information regarding permissions write to author at Olivia@TheMenuAtHome.com
Reviewers may quote brief passages in review.

Please note that credit for the images used in this book go to the respective owners. You can view this at:
TheMenuAtHome.com/image-list

Olivia Rogers
TheMenuAtHome.com

Table of Contents

Introduction 4

Chapter 1: Juicing Truths and Myths 6

Chapter 2: Increased Fruit and Vegetable Consumption of Juicing 8

Chapter 3: Various Types of Juicers 9

Chapter 4: Centrifugal Juicers 11

Chapter 5: Masticating Juicers 13

Chapter 6: Factors to Consider When Buying Juicers ... 15

Chapter 7: Taking Care of Your Juicer 19

Chapter 8: Necessary Accessories for Juicing 21

Chapter 9: The Importance of Juicing Organic 23

Chapter 10: Produce not Suitable for Juicing 25

Chapter 11: Parts of Produce Your Juicer Won't Like ... 26

Chapter 12: Extending the Life of the Juice 28

Chapter 13: Best Fruits for Juicing 30

Chapter 14: The Best Berries for Juicing and for General Health 33

Chapter 15: Best Vegetables for Juicing 35

Final Words 37

Disclaimer 39

Introduction

For your body to be healthy and functional it needs a certain amount of vitamins and minerals. Juicing is one of the best ways to give the body the nutrients it needs to function optimally. Countless cultures have collected easy to find fruits, such as pomegranates, oranges and lemons, and used them to make beverages.

The Essenes, a desert tribe in ancient Israel, pounded pomegranates and figs into a fine mash that provided subtle form and profound strength. Passion fruit was used in ancient Peru in combination with water to make a refreshing drink. So, juicing is not some latest fad of the last couple of decades.

Juicing was introduced into the modern age by Dr. Norman W. Walker, who published his book "Raw Vegetables Juices" in 1936. These days the benefits of fresh juice are well-known, and the importance of juicing is on the rise because of our modern diet.

The diet most people follow is not the healthy natural diet our ancestors followed. Commercial methods of farming have robbed the soil from vital minerals and this means the vegetables and fruits lack minerals and vitamins.

Dr. Linus Pauling, who is a famous Nobel Prize winner, blamed minerals deficiencies in the diet and the soil for most of the illnesses, diseases and ailments. There is no secret that in most places the crops are raised in toxic soil and laced with commercial crop fertilizers. Farm animals are raised in unsanitary and brutal conditions, many of the foods that are grown have been genetically altered, and livestock are feed steroids to make them produce more meat and so on. It is also well-known that the world's seafood supply has been contaminated in large parts with environmental poisons.

The average American consumes less than 20 different kinds of foods and if you combine this with packaging and storage, overcooking, shipping procedures of various countries, the processing and refinement of food, then the it is practically impossible for the average person to get enough nutrients. Juicing is the best way to provide your body with a wide spectrum of nutrients because it condenses many different varieties of produce into one single glass.

Chapter 1: Juicing Truths and Myths

If you are a beginner and are maybe still a bit unsure about the effectiveness and usefulness of juicing, then it is necessary to clear some of the smoke and bust some myths about juicing. There are people who claim that juicing is just a waste of money, energy and time, and that eating whole fruits is a much better option.

Of course, raw fruits and vegetables are very nutritious but due to the fiber content of whole fruits and vegetables, the nutrients also take more time and be absorbed and assimilated.

90% of the antioxidants on fruits are in the juice, not in the fiber, according to the Department of Agriculture. It is practically impossible and unpractical for people to get enough nutrients from eating raw vegetables and fruits. A person can get more nutrients from one single glass of juice than several servings of fruit and vegetables.

It is also important to keep in mind that many of the produce also goes through lots of abuse before being put into a bottle or can.

For example, when vegetables and fruits and frozen as concentrates then the chemical processes destroy a large portion of the enzymes and nutrients. So, they cannot be compared to juice made from fresh ingredients.

Read This FIRST - 100% FREE BONUS

FOR A LIMITED TIME ONLY – Get Olivia's best-selling book *"The #1 Cookbook: Over 170+ of the Most Popular Recipes Across 7 Different Cuisines!"* absolutely FREE!

Readers have absolutely loved this book because of the wide variety of recipes. It is highly recommended you check these recipes out and see what you can add to your home menu!

Once again, as a big thank-you for downloading this book, I'd like to offer it to you *100% FREE for a LIMITED TIME ONLY!*

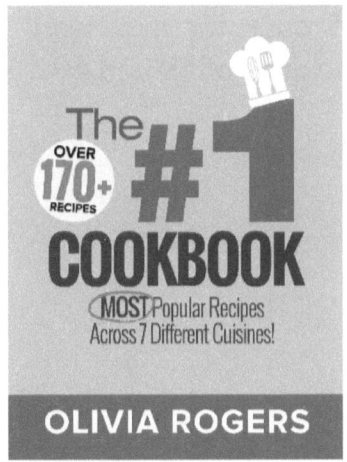

Get your free copy at:

TheMenuAtHome.com/Bonus

Chapter 2: Increased Fruit and Vegetable Consumption of Juicing

Juicing helps people consume more vegetables and fruits. To make 6-8 ounces of fresh carrot juice, it takes half a pound of carrots. According to an article published in September 2006 in the "Journal of the American Dietetic Association", most Americans consume well under the daily recommended level of fruits and vegetables.

One cup of fresh fruit or one cup of 100% fruit juice equals one serving of fruit. The ChooseMyPlate.gov guidelines of U.S. Department of Agriculture recommend 2 cups of fruits per day for men between the ages of 19 and 30 and 1.5 cups for women aged 31 and older; 2 cups for women 51 and older; 2, 5 cups for men aged 51 and older and women between the ages of 19 and 50.

Chapter 3: Various Types of Juicers

Juicing is very simple, fast and convenient but if you want to create high quality beverages then it certainly would pay off to learn the ins and outs of juicing and to invest a bit more money in a quality juicer.

Before you hastily buy a juicer, you first need to learn how to best take care of your juicer, so it lasts as much as possible, what produce is best for juicing and what is not, what types of juicers do you actually need, what accessories you need and don't need. Doing this type of homework pays off.

Basically, a juicer is mechanical devices that can be operated either electrically or manually. It is designed to extract juice from leafy greens, fruits and vegetables. What type of juicer you ultimately buy for yourself is up to you, but it is important to be aware of the different types of juicers that are on the market.

There are different types of juicers for different purposes:

- Centrifugal juicers
- Masticating juicers
- Triturating juicers
- Wheatgrass juicers
- Citrus juicers

- Manual juicers

Chapter 4: Centrifugal Juicers

Centrifugal juicers are the most popular types of juicers because they are the cheapest, oldest and have a simple design with a shredder and a strainer. The produce is shredded by a spinning basket after which the juice is forced through a fine strainer the force of the centrifuge.

The Advantage of Centrifugal Juicers

- The juice output is really fast due to the high speed and this makes the centrifugal juicer ideal for juicing on a large scale.

- There is very little preparation required because it is easy to put together and to use.

- It is inexpensive when compared to other types and models, which makes it ideal for beginners.

- This type of juicer can easily be found in department and electrical stores everywhere.

- Preparation time can also be cut short by feeding whole produce into the large and wide feeding chute.

The Disadvantages of Centrifugal Juicers

- Centrifugal juicers generally have only a 1-2-year warranty.

- The juice separates easily because it consists mainly of water.

- The juice cannot be stored for longer periods of time because the quick oxidation does not allow it.

- The yield of this type of juicers is quite low because it is not a very efficient way of juicing.

- Centrifugal juicer does not juice wheatgrass, herbs or leafy greens very well either.

- The juice itself has quite a bit of foam due to the high rate of speed that traps the air.

- Because the blades do not penetrate the produce deep enough, some of the minerals, vitamins and enzymes are not extracted from the produce.

- The motor makes lots of noise as well.

There is a bit more disadvantages than advantages, but this does not mean you should not get a centrifugal juicer. It is possible to get a good quality juicer for fewer than 100 dollars and this is often the first juicer beginners buy and there is really no need to dish out lots of money for a more expensive juicer that just sits in the closet.

Once you have got the hang of juicing and have used the centrifugal juicer for some time then you can think about getting a higher quality model.

Chapter 5: Masticating Juicers

Masticating juicers work with a single gear or an auger, which is like a drill bit and with the auger comes a rotating helical screw that acts as a screw conveyor to remove the leftover pulp. The juice which is extracted from the pulp is then collected and strained through a wire mesh.

The produce inside is crushed and squeezed against the walls of the juicer once the auger starts to turn. The leftover juice is forced out and the screen, filter and wire mesh that are lined in the sides of the walls keep hold of the pulp.

Because the masticating juicers operate at a slower pace, the juice extract is not heated up and this means that much more of the vital nutrients and enzymes are left intact. A person can enjoy a more nutrient-rich juice by using the masticating type juicer.

The benefits of masticating juicers!

- The yield of the produce from fruits and vegetables is much higher because of the slower turning auger. The pulp of masticating juicers is much drier, which is a sign that the yield is higher. Results show that masticating type juicers produce about 15-20% more juice than do centrifugal type juicers.

- The enzymes, nutrients and trace minerals are not exposed to the heat of masticating juicers. The crushing and chewing mechanisms of this process means less foam on top of the juice and a healthier juicer for you.

- Masticating type juicers are effective and also efficient in juicing a variety of produce. They can effortlessly juice leaves, leafy greens, various fruits and vegetables as well. By using that type of juicer, you can also juice spinach, celery, wheatgrass, parsley, various herbs and other things effectively.

- These types of juicers are also versatile because the process of making juice allows a person to homogenize foods and make butter, ice-cream, sorbets, baby foods, sauces, pates and more. Some models are also able to make bread sticks and pastas for example. Due to the slower speed the masticating juicer is also more likely to last longer.

Chapter 6: Factors to Consider When Buying Juicers

Besides the cost difference there are lots of factors to consider when buying a juicer. To be able to make the right choice, a person needs to consider all of these factors very carefully and only then make a decision.

- **Ease of Use**

    If you are a beginner and are looking to get your first taste of making your own juices, then look for a juicer that does not require much effort and time to operate and to clean. Juicing enthusiasts are willing to spend more time on juicing but if you are just starting out then ease of use is a real plus.

- **Reliability**

    If you are on the market for a juicer then check out some of the customer reviews, especially when it comes to reliability. Some juicers break down easily, which requires you to change parts and that is a real hassle.

- **Multiple Speeds**

    It would be best to buy a juicer that has at least 2 speeds – slower speed for easier produce and higher speed for tougher produce. Cheap models only tend to have one speed. Also make sure that your juicer has electronic circuitry that maintains blade speed during juicing.

- **Horsepower**

To avoid burning out; make sure that your juicer has at least half a horsepower.

- **Feed Tube**

Some juicers have a really small feeding tubes and this means you need to cut the produce into smaller pieces. To avoid this, make sure that the feeding tube of your juicer is large and also make sure the tube is easy and comfortable to use for you.

- **Output**

Obviously, you would want to get as much juice out of the pulp as possible. So, make sure that you check out the amount of juice a specific model can extract from a given quantity of produce. Ideally you would want to have a juicer that extracts at least 90% of the juice out of the pulp. Generally, the juicers that collect the pulp to an outside collector leave less pulp behind than those that collect the pulp inside the machine.

- **Versatility**

It is also important to be able to juice a large variety of produce, such as pineapple skins, carrots, beets, and watermelon rinds, delicate greens like parsley, lettuce and herbs.

- **Size**

It is also important to buy the right size of juicer for your specific needs. When you plan to make juice just for your own needs then choose a juicer with a beaker that holds a cup.

- **Simplicity**

The fewer parts juicers have the fewer parts there are to clean as well. Quite a few really good juicers have lots of parts and since the juicer needs to be washed properly after juicing then it can be a real disadvantage. It can also take some time to reassemble the juicer as well. Centrifugal juicers tend to be easier to wash than masticating juicers. Of course, you need to make sure that your juicer is dishwasher safe.

- **Continuous Juicing**

It would be better to choose a machine that does not eject the pulp into center basket but rather collects into a receptacle. When a juicer has a center basket then it means you need to stop the machine and wash out the basket to be able to continue juicing.

- **Quality**

It is also crucial to ensure that your juicer is securely and solidly on your counter when you use it, otherwise you can find lots of juice on the floor.

- **Noise**

    Obviously, the quieter a juicer is the better. Some brands and types are very loud, and you might even need to wear earplugs when using them. More expensive models and centrifugal juicers tend to be on the quiet side.

Chapter 7: Taking Care of Your Juicer

Every home appliance that is used frequently experiences wear and tear. If you want to make your juicer last for as long as possible then you need to respect its limitations, size, quirks, keep it in good working order and keep it clean as well. It is always better to be safe than sorry when dealing with machinery that has sharp blades and motors.

Here are a few tips and trade secrets to ensure smooth juicing:

- Carefully wash all of the produce before juicing. Remove mold, bruises, dings and blemishes.

- Go organic whenever possible. Organic produce is certainly more expensive, but it also means you don't have to peel everything before placing the produce into the juicer and lose out of the nutrients. Non-organic produce is sprayed with pesticides that penetrate the skins, which is the largest source of nutrients in the produce.

- Always make sure you peel tangerines, oranges, bananas, pineapples, kiwifruits and grapefruits, even if they are organic.

- The leaves and stems of many produce, such as small grape stems, strawberry caps, beet stems and leaves, contain higher concentration of nutrients. So, it is best not to take them all out.

- Cut most of the produce into sections and strips that can easily fit into your juicer tube without having to jam or force them in. Of course, with experience you will learn what size works best.

- To catch the pulp during juicing, make sure you insert a grocery store-sized plastic bag in the pulp receptacle of your juicer. The pulp can be used for composting; cooking or you can just throw it away.

Chapter 8: Necessary Accessories for Juicing

On top of a quality juicer, you might also need some basic equipment that you already might have in your house. Having sharp knives for peeling, coring and chopping is certainly needed. So, if you don't have sharp knives then it would be wise to make the investment.

It is also important to buy a stiff brush to be able to scrub vegetables such as carrots and beets. Having a high-quality peeler in hand is also a big plus because it allows removing the least amount of skin possible. This ensures that you are not peeling away the essential nutrients found under the skin.

There are also other accessories that make juicing much easier and comfortable. It is good to have a sieve for straining juices, flexible rubber spatulas, measuring cups and spoons. To avoid transferring any potentially dangerous bacteria into your juice, make sure you use plastic instead of wood.

Utensils, cutter boards and counter tops and many other types of equipment come into direct contact with fresh produce and therefore they need to be washed thoroughly with hot water and soap. Also use a mild bleach solution to rinse and sanitize them. Peeled and cut fruits and vegetables should be placed on a separate clean plate and avoid adding them back on top of the cutting board.

If you have been using a wooden cutting board then it would be time to replace it with a heavy plastic cutting board that can easily fit into your dishwasher. Cutting boards that are made out of wood are porous and absorb bacteria and also allow it to grow. The same is with sponges that soak up the bacteria.

Chapter 9: The Importance of Juicing Organic

Use organic vegetables and fruits for juicing whenever possible because organic produce is grown without the use of chemical biocides and synthetic fertilizers. For example, the conventional U.S. agricultural industry goes through over 1 billion pounds of herbicides and pesticides each year.

Only about 2% of this amount kills the insects; the remaining 98% goes into the air, soil, food supply and water – this includes nonorganic fruits and vegetables that people eat. So, if you buy and consume organic produce then you circumvent this health hazard.

When looking for organic produce in the store or market, look for labels that marked "certified" organic. When this label is attached to the food then this means the produce has been grown according to the strict standards of the National Organic Program. These standards include the inspection of processing facilities and farms, testing the soil and water for pesticides, detailed record keeping and so on.

Certain produces are especially vulnerable to pesticide contamination, which is another reason to buy organic. These produces includes apricots, apples, cherries, bell peppers, grapes, celery, cucumbers, green beans, strawberries, green beans, peaches and spinach.

It is also best to avoid using produce that has been irradiated or subjected to gamma ray radiation to kill germs and pests and to prolong the shelf life of produce. Irradiation can lead to the formation of certain chemicals in the produce called radiolytic products that include benzene and formaldehydes.

It has to be pointed out that although the FDA has approved irradiation, then the average dose that is used to decontaminate certain produce has been measured at levels of 5 million times what a person would receive during a chest x-ray.

This radiation is dangerous, and it also kills of minerals and vitamins. Not to mention that irradiating vegetables and fruits also releases a great deal of harmful free radicals.

Chapter 10: Produce not Suitable for Juicing

The fact is that not every fruit and vegetable – or even every part of every vegetable and fruit – lends itself for juicing.

For example, produce that have low water content are not very suitable for juicing. This includes bananas and avocados. Of course, you can still use them in your juice, but you need to run them through the juicer by itself before adding them to the main juice.

Produce that do not give much in terms of yield are also not ideal for juicing. There are certain fruits that do not separate very well from their pulp: coconut, papaya, cantaloupe, strawberries, peach, honeydew, prunes and plums for example. When you want to juice these type of produce then juice them separately and add them later to the juicer mixture.

Chapter 11: Parts of Produce Your Juicer Won't Like

There are also lots of parts of different produce that cannot be juiced very well. This includes categories of stems, leaves and skins of otherwise juiceable produce that should not be part of your juice.

This includes:

- The peels of grapefruit, oranges, nectarines and tangerines contain bitter oils that can cause digestive problems for some people. Lime and lemon peels can be juiced however if they are organic.

- It is important to remove the stones, pits and hard seeds from plums, peaches, cherries, apricots and mangoes. They are just too big for most juicers to handle and can easily cause damage to your juicer. Other seeds that are softer, such as seeds from lemons, oranges, grapes, tangerines, watermelons and cantaloupes won't damage the juicer.

- Seeds from apples contain tiny amounts of cyanide, a poison that can cause problems for the elderly, children and some adults that suffer from food sensitivity.

- The peels of papayas and mangos contain irritants that can be harmful when they are consumed in large quantities.

- Rhubarb greens and carrots are bitter and contain toxic substances.

- The juicer blades can be dulled when juicing large stems from grapes.

- You should not juice the peels of any produce that is grown in a foreign country where carcinogenic pesticides are legal.

- I don't have to mention that any produce that has splotches, bruises, dings and molds should not be juiced. To get a high-quality juice make sure that all the produce is freshly washed, free of any kind of blemishes and scrubbed free of dirt.

- It is also not ideal to use dried fruits, such as raisins and figs. If you really want to use figs, then make sure you soak them for 8-10 hours in water.

Chapter 12: Extending the Life of the Juice

Juice is something that is fragile and spoils rather fast. To get the most out of the juice in terms of vitamins and minerals you need to drink it right away. The juice spoils in just 24 hours, even when the juice is refrigerated.

If you are unable to consume your homemade juice right away then store the juice in the refrigerator in an opaque, airtight and insulated container. Air, heat and light will quickly turn the juice brown and zap all of the nutrients.

If you are unable to find fresh fruit for juicing, then you can also substitute dry-packing frozen fruits without added sugars from your local supermarket. Some of the fresh taste and nutrients can be lost but most of them will remain intact when the produce is dry-packed.

It is also a good idea to buy large quantities of fruits and vegetables when they are locally available and freeze them for your own personal use. Drinking juice made out of frozen fruits is certainly better than drinking no juice at all.

The best way to freeze fruits is to clean, slice, peel and section fruits into smaller pieces about the size of an inch that are spread out across the baking sheet, covered with plastic and added into the freezer until frozen. Transfer the fruit into a heavy, resealable plastic bag, write down the date and make sure you use them within 2 months.

Frozen fruit can be used for juicing but canned fruit is not ideal for sure. Canned produce tends to be soft and mushy, and the fruit in cans is full of sugars or packed in sugary syrup. You should never store or refrigerate the juice of cabbages, melons and cruciferous vegetables but rather drink the juice right away or toss the left-over juice away.

Chapter 13: Best Fruits for Juicing

All kinds of fruits, whether they are grown in the ground, grown on trees or on bushes, are full nutrients and acids that heal, strengthen and cleanse the body. Fruits, also known as body cleansers, contain both complex and simple carbohydrates and they release energy over an extended time period.

Below is a list of some of the more popular fruits that people like to use for juicing purpose:

- **Apples**

    They are rich in B-vitamins, vitamin C, vitamin A, biotin, folic acid and loads of beneficial minerals that support healthy hair, skin and nails. Apples also contain pectin, which is a special fiber that absorbs toxins, helps to reduce cholesterol and stimulates digestion. Apples are very versatile, and this makes them very easy to blend with other juices. Apples yield about 6-8 ounces of juice per pound.

- **Apricots**

    They are high in vitamin A and beta-carotene. They are also good sources of potassium and fiber. They yield about 6 ounces of juice per pound.

- **Cherries**

Rich in vitamin B, vitamin A, vitamin C, niacin, folic acid and loads of minerals. Cherries reduce the acidity of the blood because they are potent alkalizers. Due to this, cherries are used for prostate disorders, arthritis and gout. Cherries yield about 6-8 ounces of juice per pound.

- **Grapefruit**

They are rich in potassium, phosphorus, calcium, vitamin C. The red and pink varieties of grapefruits are less acidic and sweeter than white grapes. Grapefruits help to reduce skin colds, ear disorders, fever, strengthen capillary walls, heal bruising, indigestion, scurvy, varicose veins, obesity, and morning sickness. The yield is 6-8 ounces per pound.

- **Lemons**

They are high in vitamin C and citric acid. Lemons have great antibacterial properties and they are high in antioxidants. They also relieve reduce anemia, blood disorders, constipation, ear disorders, gout, colds, sore throats, skin infections, indigestion, scurvy, skin infections, and obesity. The yield is about 4-5 ounces of juice per pound.

- **Oranges**

Rich sources of vitamin B, K, C, folic acid, amino acids, biotin and minerals. Oranges strengthen capillary walls, benefit the heart and lungs and cleanse the gastrointestinal track. They help to reduce lung disorders, skin disorders, pneumonia, rheumatism, scurvy, anemia, blood disorders, colds, fever, heart disease, high blood pressure and liver disorders. The yield is about 6-8 ounces per pound.

Chapter 14: The Best Berries for Juicing and for General Health

- **Cranberries**

  High in vitamin B complex, vitamin C, folic acid and vitamin A. Cranberries are useful because they help to keep the bacteria from clinging to the wall of the bladder, which in turn helps to prevent bladder infections. Cranberries are also used for treating disorders of the kidney, urinary tract and lungs, and skin disorders, asthma, diarrhea, fever, fluid retention and they facilitate weight loss. The yield is 4-6 ounces per pound.

- **Blackberries and Blueberries**

  Both of these are full of sapronins that help to improve heart health. These berries also contain minerals, vitamins C, disease-fighting antioxidants and phytochemicals. The yield is 3 ounces of juice per pound.

- **Raspberries**

  They are full of vitamin C, potassium and contain 64 calories per cup. The yield is 4-5 ounces per pound.

- **Strawberries**

  They are packed with calcium, iron, vitamin C, folate, magnesium and potassium – all of which are vital for the proper functioning of the immune system and for strong connective tissues. The yield is 4-5 ounces per pound.

Chapter 15: Best Vegetables for Juicing

- **Broccoli**

    Packed with fiber and also protein. It is loaded with antioxidants, calcium, vitamin C, B6 and vitamin E. It is generally used in combination with other juices because the taste is quite strong. The yield is 6 ounces per pound.

- **Cabbage**

    Cabbages come in many varieties, from white to green, red and Savoy cabbage. All of the members of the cabbage family are high in vitamin B6, vitamin C and vitamin A. The yield is 6 ounces per pound.

- **Beets**

    Both the beetroots and beet greens are highly nutritious and judicable. The roots of beets are full of potassium, calcium, vitamin C and vitamin A. The yield per pound is 6-7 ounces.

- **Carrots**

    The ultimate vegetables for juicing. Carrots give a sweet and mild taste to various juice combos and it also tastes great by itself. Carrots are full of vitamins B, A, E, D, C and K. They are also high in sodium, potassium, phosphorus, calcium and various trace minerals. Fresh carrot juice helps to improve hair, digestion, skin and nails. The juice also has a diuretic effect and cleanses the liver. The yield is 6-8 ounces per pound.

There are also many other fantastic vegetables that can be used for juicing: radishes, potatoes, Parsnips, ginger, garlic, fennel, celery, yams and sweet potatoes, green onions, turnips, tomatoes, string beans, bell peppers, summer squash and more.

Final Words

I would like to thank you for downloading my book and I hope I have been able to help you and educate you about something new.

If you have enjoyed this book and would like to share your positive thoughts, could you please take 30 seconds of your time to go back and give me a review on my Amazon book page!

I greatly appreciate seeing these reviews because it helps me share my hard work!

Again, thank you and I wish you all the best with your cooking journey!

Last Chance to Get YOUR Bonus!

FOR A LIMITED TIME ONLY – Get Olivia's best-selling book *"The #1 Cookbook: Over 170+ of the Most Popular Recipes Across 7 Different Cuisines!"* absolutely FREE!

Readers have absolutely loved this book because of the wide variety of recipes. It is highly recommended you check these recipes out and see what you can add to your home menu!

Once again, as a big thank-you for downloading this book, I'd like to offer it to you *100% FREE for a LIMITED TIME ONLY!*

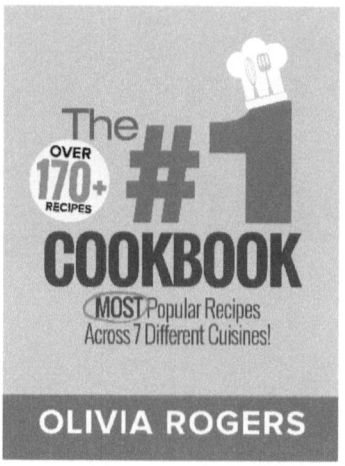

Get your free copy at:

TheMenuAtHome.com/Bonus

Disclaimer

This book and related site provides recipe and food advice in an informative and educational manner only, with information that is general in nature and that is not specific to you, the reader. The contents of this book and related site are intended to assist you and other readers in your personal efforts. Consult your physician or nutritionist regarding the applicability of any information provided in our information to you.

Nothing in this book should be construed as personal advice or diagnosis, and must not be used in this manner. The information provided about conditions is general in nature. This information does not cover all possible uses, actions, precautions, side-effects, or interactions of medicines, or medical procedures. The information in this site should not be considered as complete and does not cover all diseases, ailments, physical conditions, or their treatment.

No Warranties: The authors and publishers don't guarantee or warrant the quality, accuracy, completeness, timeliness, appropriateness or suitability of the information in this book, or of any product or services referenced by this site.

The information in this site is provided on an "as is" basis and the authors and publishers make no representations or warranties of any kind with respect to this information. This site may contain inaccuracies, typographical errors, or other errors.

Liability Disclaimer: The publishers, authors, and other parties involved in the creation, production, provision of information, or delivery of this site specifically disclaim any responsibility, and shall not be held liable for any damages, claims, injuries, losses, liabilities, costs, or obligations including any direct, indirect, special, incidental, or consequences damages (collectively known as "Damages") whatsoever and howsoever caused, arising out of, or in connection with the use or misuse of the site and the information contained within it, whether such Damages arise in contract, tort, negligence, equity, statute law, or by way of other legal theory.

www.ingramcontent.com/pod-product-compliance
Lightning Source LLC
Chambersburg PA
CBHW021134080526
44587CB00012B/1288